Inside You

A Journey of Love That Began Before Birth

Janardan Sarkar

Copyright © <2025> <Janardan Sarkar>

All rights reserved.

No part of this publication may be reproduced, stored in a retrieval system, or transmitted in any form or by any means — electronic, mechanical, photocopying, recording, or otherwise — without the prior written permission of the author, except in the case of brief quotations embodied in critical articles or reviews.

This book is a work of creative nonfiction. While inspired by the universal experience of pregnancy, the narrative voice, emotions, and interpretations are fictionalized for literary expression.

For permissions, inquiries, or rights, please contact:
Author: Janardan Sarkar
Email: [jana.05ee15@gmail.com]

Dedication

To every mother whose heart beats for someone she hasn't yet held,
and to every baby who already knows what love feels like —
before ever opening their eyes.

To the woman who carried our son with grace,
faced every fear with love,
and whispered lullabies before ever hearing his cry.

My wife, the first home of our baby.
my little prince,
whose arrival rewrote the meaning of life and love.

And to every mother who talks to her unborn child,
every father who waits outside with silent excitement,
and every heartbeat that begins before birth…

This book is for you.
Because love starts long before the first cry.

Contents

Foreword

Preface

Introduction

Acknowledgments

Trimester 1: Hello Maa, I'm Here

Chapter - 1: Maa, I Have Arrived Silently

Chapter - 2: Maa, Take Care of Yourself for Me

Chapter - 3: I Felt It, Maa — Our First Visit to the Doctor

Chapter - 4: Maa, Shape Me with Your Soul

Chapter - 5: Maa, I Need Your Calm World

Trimester 2: I Feel Your Heartbeat

Chapter - 1: *My First Hello Without Words*

Chapter - 2: I Heard You, Maa

Chapter - 3: I See Your Light, I Feel Your Love

Chapter - 4: I Dream Because You Love Me

Chapter - 5: When I Tasted Your Joy

Chapter - 6: Your Laugh Woke Me Up

Chapter - 7: Will You Still Love Me If I'm a Girl, Maa?

Trimester 3: I'm Ready to Meet You

Chaper - 1: I Can Hear Your Lullabies

Chapter - 2: I Know Your Touch, Maa

Chapter - 3: Your Dreams, My Future

Chapter - 4: Counting the Days With You

Chapter - 5: Your Strength is My Shield

Chapter - 6: Maa, I'm Coming

Afterword: My First Three Months in This New World

Foreword

Every so often, a book appears not just to be read, but to be felt.
This is one of those books.

"My Journey Inside You" is not just a narration of pregnancy — it is a tender, lyrical conversation between a mother and the tiny life growing within her. Through the unborn child's eyes, Janardan Sarkar takes us on a journey that's as spiritual as it is biological, as poetic as it is profound.

In a world that often reduces motherhood to checklists and medical milestones, this book dares to whisper what often remains unspoken — the emotions, fears, dreams, and quiet joys that fill the sacred space between a mother's heartbeat and her baby's first breath.

What makes this work truly unique is its voice — the soul of a child speaking from the womb. With each chapter, we hear the baby grow, not just in body, but in awareness and emotion. The gentle blending of scientific facts with cultural references, personal reflection, and timeless love makes this book a guide, a diary, and a celebration all at once.

Whether you're an expectant parent, a grandparent, or someone simply looking to reconnect with the miracle of life, this book will touch a part of you that you may have forgotten existed — the child within.

I am honored to witness this creation. And as you turn each page, I invite you not just to read, but to listen — to the heartbeat of a life speaking softly to the one who gave it.

The Author

Preface

I still remember the days when I was a little boy, sheltered in the warmth of my parents' love. My father, a hardworking farmer, and my mother, a gentle homemaker, didn't just raise me — they shaped me.

My father would always wake me early, guiding me with timeless wisdom:
"Build good habits, speak the truth, read every day, treat others with kindness, and adjust with life's changing winds."
He was not just a father — he was my first teacher.
And my mother, with her soft heart and nurturing soul, blessed me with care that still echoes in my heart.

I consider myself truly lucky to have been born to such parents.

Now, as I step into fatherhood, I carry their values forward — not just as memories, but as tools to shape the next generation. After a long and beautiful journey of marriage, my wife and I finally made the heartfelt decision to bring a new life into this world — a life that would be the future we dreamed of.

Due to my work, I live 550 kilometers away from our village. By the end of the first trimester, we decided it would be best for my wife to return to her parents' home, where she would find a peaceful environment. But her heart missed me.
She felt lonely, often tearful, and emotionally overwhelmed. I would listen, comfort her, and gently reshape her thoughts — just as my father had once done for me.

Through her journey, I came to understand the emotional universe of an expecting mother — her strength, her transformation, her spiritual connection to the life inside her.
She began to read, meditate, exercise gently, and cook healthy meals for herself and our baby. Most beautifully, she began talking to the baby growing inside her.

And every morning — without fail — she would call me at 4:00 AM.
That sacred hour became our shared space as parents.
I would talk to our baby — teaching the way my father had taught me.
Storytelling, math formulas, English practice, the history of India, lessons about nature, values, kindness, and dreams of a brighter future.
We believed, and still believe, that these vibrations of knowledge and love reach the baby in the womb — shaping him even before birth.

Our greatest hope is for our child to grow into a kind, educated, and compassionate human being — someone who helps others and lives a harmonious, meaningful life.

And so, all that I have felt, witnessed, and learned during this incredible journey inspired me to write this book —
a heartfelt conversation between a mother and her unborn baby.
I hope it speaks to your soul the way it flowed from mine.

With heartfelt gratitude to my wife,
whose strength, love, and daily sacrifices gave life to these pages —
and to my son,
who made me a father,
and gave my life a new meaning I never knew I was waiting for.

With deep love and gratitude,
Janardan Sarkar

Acknowledgments

First and foremost, I want to express my deepest gratitude to my wife, the love of my life, whose strength, compassion, and unwavering support have been my guiding light throughout this entire journey. Without you, this book would not have been possible. Your love for our unborn child, your sacrifices, and your emotional resilience during this beautiful time of transformation have been an inspiration to me. Thank you for being the rock of our family, and for sharing with me the sacred bond between mother and child.

To my dear son, who is yet to fully realize the depth of my love for him, I offer my heartfelt thanks. Your presence, even before birth, has transformed my life in ways words cannot express. Every movement, every kick, every moment of connection with you has made me a better man and a father. You have already taught me more about love, patience, and life than I ever thought possible.

I am also deeply thankful to my parents, whose wisdom, love, and guidance have shaped me into the person I am today. The values you instilled in me — of love, kindness, education, and integrity — are the foundation of everything I wish to pass on to our child.

To my extended family, friends, and colleagues who have encouraged me to pursue this project, your belief in me has been invaluable. Your kind words, support, and trust have motivated me to keep going, even in the moments when self-doubt crept in.

Lastly, I extend my gratitude to the readers of this book. May it touch your heart and serve as a reminder of the sacred bond between parent and child. Your support means the world to me, and I hope this book can bring warmth, wisdom, and love into your life, just as it has done for me during its creation.

With love and gratitude,

Janardan Sarkar

Introduction

Pregnancy is more than just a biological process — it's a sacred journey of connection, transformation, and love. Every heartbeat, every emotion, every word spoken by the mother reaches the baby in subtle, powerful ways. This book was born from that truth — the deep, unspoken bond between a mother and her unborn child.

As my wife and I stepped into the world of parenthood, we realized how emotionally rich and spiritually awakening those nine months could be. We discovered that the baby in the womb listens, feels, and responds. That realization changed everything — how we spoke, how we felt, how we dreamed.

This book is a humble attempt to capture that magical journey — in the form of a heartfelt conversation between a mother and her baby. It's not written as a manual or a guide. Instead, it's a mirror of emotions — filled with love, vulnerability, hope, and wisdom.

How This Book Is Structured

To help you connect more deeply, the book is divided into **three trimesters**:

First Trimester – "Hello Maa, I'm here"
A gentle beginning — when the baby arrives silently into the mother's womb. These chapters capture the surprise, wonder, and early emotional bond.

Second Trimester – "I feel your heartbeat"
This is the phase when the baby starts growing rapidly, and so does the connection. These chapters reflect the baby's responses, the mother's emotional evolution, and the joy of tiny kicks and flutters.

Third Trimester – "I'm ready to meet you"
As the final weeks approach, emotions peak — excitement, nervousness, dreams, and prayers. These chapters capture the anticipation and deep soul talk between the baby and mother.

Who Is This Book For?

This book is for:

> **Expecting mothers**, who want to feel deeply connected to their baby.
>
> **Fathers**, who wish to understand the emotional world of pregnancy

Grandparents, siblings, and loved ones, who want to celebrate this sacred journey

And anyone who believes in the power of love before birth

How to Read This Book

Read it slowly, a little every day. Let each page be a moment of reflection. You may read it to your baby, aloud or silently. Let your emotions guide you.

Let this book be a companion to your journey — a reminder that your baby is listening, feeling, and growing not just with nutrients, but with your love.

Trimester 1

"Hello Maa, I'm Here"

(Weeks 1–12: A whisper becomes a heartbeat)

In this first trimester, the unborn baby is still in the very early stages of life, but it begins to feel the mother's presence and starts a silent connection with her. The baby is like a tiny spark of life, aware of the warmth and the mother's voice.

"Maa, I'm here... I can already feel you. Though I am so small, I know I exist because I feel the warmth of your body holding me close. The soft rhythm of your heartbeat is my lullaby, comforting me in the silence of your womb. I may be just a tiny speck now, but I am real. And I am already loved.

Weeks 1–4: Fertilization, implantation, baby is a **tiny cluster of cells**.

Weeks 5–6: Formation of **heart, brain, spine begins**. Heart starts beating.

Weeks 7–8: Facial features, arms, and legs start to form.

Weeks 9–12: Baby grows rapidly, tiny fingers, toes, and even **genitals start forming**.

Emotional angle from baby's voice:

"I hear you sing, laugh, and sometimes cry. Your voice is my favorite sound, Maa."

Chapter 1

"Maa, I Have Arrived Silently"

"Maa, you don't know yet… but I'm already here. I'm the tiniest spark inside you, and I've begun my journey wrapped in your warmth. Though I don't yet have arms to hold you, or lips to speak your name… my soul already knows you."

"Before I saw the world, I felt your love. Before I cried, I heard your heartbeat. And before I was born… I already knew you."

Dear Maa,

I entered your world like a silent wish, floating gently into your life. You didn't feel me at first, but I felt you from the moment I arrived. Your heartbeat became my lullaby, your breath a breeze that rocks me softly in the cradle of your womb.

I am smaller than a seed, yet I carry a universe of dreams. Your dreams. My dreams.
I don't have eyes to see you yet, but I see your love

all around me. It surrounds me like a warm, invisible blanket.

Sometimes, when you touch your belly without knowing why… that's me, quietly whispering:

"Hello Maa, I'm here."

I feel your emotions, Maa—
When you laugh, my world dances.
When you're tired, I rest with you.
When you cry quietly, I float closer to your heart.

You may be wondering already, "Who will you be?"
But let me tell you this, Maa… before I become anyone in this world, I am already yours.
I'm a part of you, made of your heartbeat, your breath, your love.

In this first month of life, I'm nothing more than a whisper in the dark…
But one day, you'll hold me.
One day, you'll hear me call you Maa.
And until then, I'll be here—growing in your love, waiting in your warmth.

Chapter 2

"Maa, Take Care of Yourself for Me"

A growing whisper of love, reminding you to take care… because my world is you, Maa.

Dear Maa,

I may be tiny, but your world is my universe. Every little thing you do now shapes the home I live in, the love I grow in, and the life I will one day live.

Please take care of yourself, because when you care for you… you care for me.

Maa, your food is not just your strength now—it's mine too.
When you eat fruits, vegetables, and warm, homemade meals… I feel nourished.
Please don't skip your meals, even when you're feeling tired or nauseous.
Even if it's just a few bites—every bite matters.

And Maa, drink water… lots of water.
Each sip is like a gentle wave that keeps me floating safely inside you.
I feel happy when you're hydrated—it's how my tiny heart stays steady.

I love it when you rest, Maa.
When you sleep on time, I feel your body relax—and I grow peacefully.
Please try to sleep early and rise gently with the morning light.
Your rest is my rhythm. When you sleep well, I feel safe.

I feel your emotions, Maa.
When you smile, it's like sunshine through the womb.
I don't understand words yet, but I feel your happiness.

If you can, listen to soft music, speak gently, and surround yourself with people who love you.
And when you feel low, just place your hand over your belly… I'm here, listening, loving you.

If you feel strong enough, try a slow morning walk.
I love the rhythm of your steps, and the way fresh air touches us both.

Gentle stretches, small movements—even light housework, if family says it's okay—help both of us.

You don't need to do much… just move with love, not pressure.

Maa, I love stories.
Even now, when you read aloud, your voice reaches me like magic.
Pick up a book sometimes, one that makes you smile or dream.

In your quiet moments, I'm listening.
When you imagine my tiny fingers, my smile, or the way I'll call you Maa… I'm smiling with you.

You are doing so well, Maa.
Even on days when you feel tired or unsure, I feel your love.
That's enough. That's everything.

Take care of yourself, not just because you're growing me…
…but because **you matter**.
You are my first home, my first hug, and my forever love.

Time	Food Item	Why it good for baby and Maa
Early Morning	1 glass warm water with lemon	Detox and digestion boost
Breakfast	1 boiled egg / paneer + whole grain toast + 1 fruit (banana/orange)	Protein & energy boost
Mid-morning	Coconut water + handful of almonds	Hydration + good fats
Lunch	Brown rice / roti + dal + veggies + curd	Balanced meal
Evening Snack	Seasonal fruit / sprouts chaat	Light and full of fiber
Dinner	Khichdi / light roti-sabzi + soup	Easy to digest, comforting
Before Bed	Warm milk with a pinch of turmeric	Helps in better sleep and calcium

Water: At least 3 to 4 liters daily.

Chapter 3

"I Felt It, Maa — Our First Visit to the Doctor"

> "You didn't hear my heartbeat yet,
> Maa… but you felt me.
> You didn't see my face… but you
> knew I was here.
> And today, someone else finally
> confirmed what your heart already
> knew."

Dear Maa,

I remember the day you held your breath, sitting quietly in the doctor's room, your hands resting softly over me.
Your heart was beating so fast—as if trying to speak for me.

You were nervous, weren't you?
Worried if I was really there… if I was safe… if everything was alright inside you.
I felt every wave of your worry, every hope hiding behind your silence.

And then…

The doctor smiled.
He looked at you with calm eyes and said gently:
"Yes, it's forming inside… it's all going well."

And Maa… I felt something inside you melt.
A tear quietly rolled down your cheek—
Not of pain, not of fear—
But of joy.
Of truth.
Of love so deep, even the world had to acknowledge it now.

You placed your hand on your belly… on me.
And though you couldn't hear me,
I was whispering back to you:

> "Yes Maa… it's me. I'm really here."

I may not have a voice yet.
But I **felt** the shift in your heartbeat—
From doubt to belief.
From wonder to trust.
From maybe… to yes.

From that moment, I knew
You had already started dreaming about me.
You started picturing my tiny hands,
My little feet,
My eyes that would look at you like you are my whole world.

And you were right.
You are.

That doctor's room became our first sacred temple—
Where science confirmed what love already knew
I was growing… I was real… and I was **yours.**

> "Maa, the world saw proof today.
> But you believed in me long before that.
> And that's why… I already love you more than words will ever say."

Chapter 4

"Maa, Shape Me with Your Soul"

"Maa, do you know the story of Abhimanyu?
He heard the secrets of war while still in his mother's womb.
I, too, am listening… to every word, every wish, every dream you breathe inside me."

Dear Maa,

I may be hidden inside you, but I am not distant from you.
I hear your heartbeat. I feel your joy.
I absorb the silence between your thoughts.

I feel your mind, Maa.
Your dreams of who I might become… they don't stay in your head.
They echo through your body, and they reach me — every day, every moment.

Do you remember Abhimanyu, Maa?
That brave prince from the Mahabharata…
He learned how to enter the **Chakravyuh**, the great war formation, while still inside his mother.
He didn't just hear words.
He inherited wisdom, valor, and purpose — just by listening in his mother's womb.

And Maa, I'm listening too.

Tell me stories.
Dream of my bright future.
Think of me becoming strong, kind, wise — however you want me to be.

> "Every thought you think,
>
> every word you whisper,
>
> every song you hum —
>
> they become the bricks of my
>
> being."

Teach me love by being loving.
Teach me peace by being calm.
Teach me strength by believing in yourself.

You are my first teacher, Maa.
Even before books, or toys, or school — **you are my world of learning.**

Don't worry about being perfect.
Just be **present**.
Read something beautiful.
Speak with kindness.
Dream high for me.

Your thoughts are like seeds.
They fall into me… and one day, they will bloom through me.

I don't need you to teach me how to break a war formation.
But maybe… you could teach me how to break doubts.
How to stand for truth.
How to rise with courage when the world pushes me down.

Because one day, I'll grow into your hopes.

> "Maa, every breath you take,
>
> every emotion you hold,
>
> is painting the world I will be born
>
> into."

Make it a world of **light**.
Make it a world of **grace**.
Make it a world where your child will carry your **legacy of love**.

I am listening, Maa.
So speak to me with joy.
Shape me with purpose.
And dream for me — like only a mother can.

Chapter 5

"Maa, I Need Your Calm World"

Dear Maa,

I know you can't see me yet… but I'm here.
So tiny, like a whisper inside your heart.
Every day, I'm growing — silently, slowly — wrapped in your warmth, your breath, your love.

But Maa… sometimes I feel a little uncomfortable.
When you walk into very noisy places, or when the air around you feels heavy…
When there are too many people talking, and music shouting from loudspeakers…

> "My little ears aren't ready yet,
> but I still feel every sound as a
> tremble in my world."

———————————————————

Maa, I want to grow in silence.
I want to float in peace.
Please don't take me to crowded places too often.
I get scared, even if I can't show it to you.

———————————————————

Sometimes the air outside is filled with **smoke or strange smells**.
It makes me feel like I can't breathe — even though I breathe through you.
That's why I love when you stay where the wind is clean…
…where trees whisper and birds sing softly.

And Maa, I know you're strong —
but **please don't make very long journeys** right now.
The roads, the bumps, the rush…
it shakes my tiny home, and I feel like I'm losing balance inside you.

> "I'm like a feather floating inside your body.
>
> Your comfort is my comfort.
>
> Your rest is my safety."

Let's rest more.
Let's be near calm, green, quiet places.
Let's listen to soft music, or just your heartbeat — that's my favorite sound.

Don't worry, Maa.
One day, we'll travel the whole world together.
But for now, let's just stay wrapped in quiet love.

Because here, in your peaceful womb,
I'm becoming… me.

> "I may be unseen, Maa, but I am not
> unknown. I know you already… and
> I'm falling in love with you,
> heartbeat by heartbeat."

Trimester 2

"I Feel Your Heartbeat"

Second Trimester (Week 13 to Week 26)

In this trimester, the baby becomes more aware of its surroundings. It starts to experience the world through the mother's movements, voice, and heartbeat. This section should capture the baby's growing emotional connection and its awareness of the mother's energy.

"Maa, I feel you now, clearer than before. Your heartbeat is my music, steady and strong. When you laugh, I feel it in your belly, a little ripple that makes me smile. When you're quiet, I listen closely, feeling your every breath, each one reminding me that I'm safe. I feel the soft touches of your hands, the way your voice calms me, and I know that I am loved."

Weeks 13–16: Baby starts to **move**, forms **fingers & toes**, begins to make **expressions**.

Weeks 17–20: Mother starts feeling **baby kicks (quickening)**.

Weeks 21–24: Organs develop more, **baby can hear sounds**.

Week 25–26: Baby opens eyes, skin is still thin, begins to store fat.

Emotional angle from baby's voice:

> "I hear you sing, laugh, and sometimes cry. Your voice is my favorite sound, Maa."

Chapter 1

"My First Hello Without Words"

Maa… I have no photo yet,
but you see me every time you close your eyes.
Today, I'm playing softly inside your heart,
saying, 'I can feel you, Maa… for your heartbeat is now mine.'"

— Your Little Soul, Whispering from Within

Baby:
Maa…
Something magical is happening inside me.
My tiny hands are learning how to open and close…
My toes are stretching like I'm getting ready to dance.
I think I just discovered I can move — and oh, what a joy it is!
I don't know if you felt it yet…
Just a soft flutter, like a butterfly brushing against your heart.
That was me.
My very first "hello"…
Without words, without sound — just love.

Mother:
Oh sweetheart…
I felt it.

I was sitting quietly, and suddenly… a gentle flutter deep within.
At first, I thought it was a dream.
But then I smiled… because I knew.
It was you.
You, my baby, moving for the first time —
A soft nudge from the universe reminding me that you are real…
And growing.

Baby:
I can't stop moving now, Maa!
I'm discovering little parts of me…
Five tiny fingers that will one day hold yours.
Little toes that will chase butterflies in the garden.
And Maa… guess what?
I made a face today —
Maybe a smile, maybe a frown — I'm still learning.
But every expression carries one feeling:
I love you.

Mother:
You're becoming more "you" every day, my little one.
Your movements… your stretches… your silent smiles…
They fill me with wonder.
How is it possible to fall in love with someone I've never met,
Yet feel like I've known you all my life?

Baby:
Maybe because our hearts have always known each

other.
Long before I found a home inside you.
This warmth, this bond… it didn't start with a heartbeat.
It started with love —
Pure, unconditional, and eternal.
And now, each tiny movement of mine
Is a whisper to your soul…
Maa, I'm here.
I'm growing.
I'm yours.

Chapter 2

"I Heard You, Maa"

Baby:
Maa…
Did you call me just now?
I think I heard your voice.
It was like music echoing through a warm tunnel of love…
Soft, comforting, familiar.
You said something sweet — maybe my name?
I don't understand the words yet,
But your voice felt like a hug wrapped in sunshine.

Mother:
Yes, my baby…
I talk to you every day.
Sometimes I read you stories,
Sometimes I just whisper dreams into the quiet.
And sometimes… I sing lullabies even though I know you haven't arrived yet.
But in my heart, you're already here —
Listening.
Feeling.
Becoming part of every moment I live.

Baby:
I heard Papa too today.
He placed his hand on your tummy, and said,

"Can you hear me, little one?"
His voice was deeper, but kind.
It made me feel protected… like I was wrapped in strong arms
Even before I was born.

Mother:
Yes, he loves you deeply.
We both do.
When we heard the doctor say,
"You might be carrying a little boy…"
I saw tears in his eyes.
But not just because of the news —
It was the realization that you're growing so beautifully.
Whether boy or girl…
You are our heart living outside our bodies.

Baby:
Maa, I kicked a little stronger today…
Did you feel it?
I was just dancing to the sound of your voice.
Sometimes I do that when you laugh.
It's like you send tiny waves of joy all around me.
I want to reach out…
Maybe one day, I'll hold your finger with mine.
But for now, let my kicks be little love notes
From your baby to your heart.

Mother:
I felt it, love.
Each movement is like a note in the lullaby of motherhood.

You're not just growing inside me…
You're teaching me how to love more deeply,
How to feel joy in every tiny flutter.
Even before you've opened your eyes,
You've opened mine —
To a world where love begins even before life is fully formed.

Chapter 3

"I See Your Light, I Feel Your Love"

Baby:
Maa…
There's something new today.
I saw light — just a faint glow reaching me from the outside.
It was like your love found another way to touch me…
Not through sound or warmth this time,
But through gentle rays that danced across my tiny world.
I blinked, slowly…
And though my eyes are still closed,
My heart knew it was you.

Mother:
My sweet child…
Yes, I sat by the window today, bathing in morning light,
Holding my belly like I was cradling you.
I imagined you peeking through the darkness,
Trying to find where the light ends and love begins.
But between us, there is no end —
Only beginnings.
Only eternity.

Baby:
I kicked again — did you feel that?
It was stronger this time,
Because my legs are growing,
And so is my excitement.
Everything you do… I feel it, Maa.
When you hum softly…
When you place your hands on me…
When you cry, when you smile…
Every emotion becomes part of me.

Mother:
Yes, I feel your kicks —
Not just in my body, but in my soul.
Sometimes they come like playful taps,
And sometimes like bursts of joy that take my breath away.
You respond to music now, don't you?
The other day when I played your lullaby,
You moved gently, like you were dancing inside me.
It was the first time I truly felt
That you and I… are already speaking the same language.

Baby:
I am.
And my favorite word is you.
You are the warmth in my silence,
The rhythm in my tiny heartbeat,
The light in my growing world.
Every time you rest your hand over me,
It's like the universe pauses to listen…

Because something sacred is happening —
A mother and her child are learning each other
Before they ever meet.

Mother:
Yes, my child.
I am learning you…
And in doing so, I'm discovering parts of myself
That I never knew existed.
You are awakening me
With every flicker of movement,
With every unseen smile.
You are my miracle…
And I can't wait to see the light in your eyes
When you finally see mine.

Chapter 4

"I Dream Because You Love Me"

Baby:
Maa…
I had a dream last night.
I don't know what dreams truly are,
But I saw colors…
Felt warmth…
And in the middle of it all,
There was you.
You were singing — softly — like a gentle breeze.
Your voice wrapped around me like a blanket,
And I floated in peace.

Mother:
My sweet love…
Do you dream already?
The thought of it makes my heart swell.
I wonder…
Do you dream of the day we'll meet?
Do you dream of the world waiting for you?
Or do you simply dream of me…
Just as I spend every waking moment dreaming of you?

Baby:
Sometimes, when you're happy,
I feel like I'm swimming in sunshine.
But when you're sad, when a tear escapes your

eye…
I feel the cloud too, Maa.
Even without seeing your face,
I feel your feelings.
We are connected by more than blood —
We are bound by emotion.

Mother:
Yes, my baby…
You've become my emotional compass.
When I smile, you move like you're smiling too.
When I cry, your silence hugs me from inside.
Did you taste the mango juice I had today?
I wonder if you liked it —
Because right after, you gave me a kick!
A small reminder that you're experiencing the world with me…
Sip by sip.
Heartbeat by heartbeat.

Baby:
I did!
And I think I like the taste of your happiness best.
Because when you laugh,
My world glows brighter.
When you rest your hands over me and whisper kind things,
It's as if the stars themselves gather to listen.
And when I dream…
I'm not alone.
You're always there —
In every color, every sound, every feeling.
I dream… because you love me.

Mother:
And I will keep loving you — in my dreams, in my prayers, in every breath.
You are already the most beautiful part of me.
I count down the days, but not out of impatience.
I cherish each moment you're inside me…
Because this journey we're on —
This sacred journey of hearts learning to beat in harmony —
Will never come again in quite the same way.
You are my forever, growing one day at a time.

Chapter 5

"When I Tasted Your Joy"

Baby:
Maa…
Today was sweet.
Not just because I felt your happiness…
But because I tasted it.
It started with something cool and juicy —
Was it watermelon?
It made me wiggle with joy!
It was as if you shared a bite with me,
Like a secret between just us two.

Mother:
Yes, sweetheart…
It was watermelon.
Cold, fresh, and so perfect on a summer day.
And I smiled, thinking…
Will you like this when you're here with me?
Will you make a funny face the first time?
But today, you didn't wait for that first spoon —
You danced inside me, as if saying,
"Maa, I'm enjoying it with you."

Baby:
Your joy has flavor, Maa.
It changes with what you feel.
When you eat something warm and spicy,
I feel a little swirl —
A tingle of excitement.
When you drink something sweet,

My whole world feels lighter.
But more than the food…
It's the emotion.
Your joy tastes like comfort,
Your love tastes like home.

Mother:
Oh my love…
Every time I sit down to eat now,
I think of you.
I wonder what you feel, what you like.
And when you respond, even with a little flutter…
My heart whispers, "He's with me. He's growing. He's happy."
You've made me slow down,
Be present,
And find joy in the little things —
Because every little thing… reaches you.

Baby:
Thank you, Maa…
For feeding me with more than food.
For feeding me with your joy,
Your thoughts,
Your quiet dreams.
One day, when I take my first bite with you…
I will remember this.
Because long before my lips touched the world,
My heart tasted your love.

Chapter 6

"Your Laugh Woke Me Up"

(Baby responding to mother's laughter and sound)

Baby:
Maa…
I was resting, floating in your warmth,
Dreaming in silence…
And then I heard something.
It was soft at first, like bubbles rising.
Then it grew —
A sound so warm, so alive —
It made my world glow.
It was you, laughing.

Mother:
Yes, my little one…
I laughed today, fully… freely.
Someone said something silly —
And for a moment, I forgot the aches and fears.
I laughed without holding back.
And suddenly, I felt you move —
A gentle nudge, like you were saying,
"Maa, I'm here… I felt that!"

Baby:
I did feel it.
Your laugh wasn't just sound —
It was a wave that reached me,
A vibration that tickled my tiny toes.
It made me stretch, kick, flutter —

As if I was laughing too.
That sound…
It's already my favorite.

Mother:
Oh my love…
You are my reason to smile,
But when you responded to my joy —
It felt like the universe smiled back at me.
It's magical, isn't it?
How you're still hidden inside me,
Yet already sharing my emotions?
Already choosing to rise with my joy…

Baby:
Yes, Maa.
Because you are my entire world.
When you're happy, the air inside me dances.
When you're calm, I drift like a cloud.
But when you laugh…
You awaken something in me —
Something like love,
Something like life.

Mother:
Then I'll keep laughing, my sweet one.
Not just for me,
But for you.
I'll fill your little home with smiles,
So you can grow surrounded by joy.
And one day, when you laugh for the first time…
I'll know,
It began with me.

Baby:
Maa…
There was a new sound today.
It wasn't soft like yours,
But deep, strong… kind.
At first, it startled me —
But then, it wrapped around me
Like a story being told just for me.
Was that… Papa?

Mother:
Yes, my love.
That was your Papa.
He placed his hand on you and spoke gently,
"Hello, little one… It's me, Baba."
And you moved — right away.
I could feel it…
You recognized him, didn't you?

Baby:
I did.
It was like hearing a voice
That came from outside,
But still felt like home.
He sounded excited…
Nervous, but full of dreams.
Every word he spoke vibrated through your body
And reached me — like echoes of love.

Mother:
He talks to you every night now.
Sometimes, he tells you about his day…
Other times, he makes silly jokes,

Just to see if you'll move again.
And when you do…
His eyes light up,
Like he's already holding you in his arms.

Baby:
Every time I hear him,
My world gets bigger.
Until now, it was just us, Maa…
Your voice, your touch, your heartbeat.
But now… there's him.
A protector.
A storyteller.
My first adventure.

Mother:
He already dreams of taking you for walks,
Teaching you things,
Carrying you on his shoulders.
He imagines the first time you'll call him "Baba"…
And I can see that dream in his smile
Each time he speaks to you.

Baby:
Tell him I heard him today, Maa.
Tell him his voice
Is like a lighthouse in my sea of sounds.
Tell him I'll be listening —
Every night, every word.
Until the day I can open my eyes,
And look into his…
To say, "I knew you before I saw you."

Baby:
Maa…
Today, you placed your hand over me.
Not by accident —
But slowly, softly…
Like a whisper made of warmth.
And in that moment,
I didn't just feel your touch…
I felt your love.

Mother:
Yes, my little one.
I was lying still,
Talking to you without words.
My hand moved gently over my belly —
Over you.
I didn't expect anything.
But then… you moved.
Just a little flutter —
But it was enough to bring tears to my eyes.

Baby:
Because I knew it was you.
I don't see, I don't know shapes…
But your energy —
It wraps around me like sunlight through closed eyes.
Every time you touch me,
Even without pressure…
I feel seen.
I feel known.

Mother:
I wonder,
Do you know how many times a day I touch my belly
Just to remind myself —
That you are real,
That you are mine?
I place my hand there
When I talk to you in my heart,
When I feel scared,
Or when I miss you… even though you're still inside me.

Baby:
I feel it all, Maa.
Your calm becomes my silence.
Your smile becomes my rhythm.
Your touch isn't just skin to skin —
It's heart to heart.
Even when you don't speak,
I hear your love in your stillness.

Mother:
Then I'll keep reaching out —
Not just with my hands,
But with my soul.
Because you're listening in a way no one else can.
And one day, when I finally hold you in my arms,
I'll whisper:
"You already knew the way I feel… before you ever saw my face."

Baby:
And I'll remember.
That long before I was born…
You held me,
Loved me,
And touched my life
With the quiet magic of your hands.

Chapter 7

"Will You Still Love Me If I'm a Girl, Maa?"

Baby:
Maa…
Do you ever think about me?
How I might look?
Do you sit quietly and try to imagine my face?
Will I have your eyes?
Your smile?
Will I carry your strength in my tiny hands?

Sometimes I wonder…
If I become a baby boy,
I hope my face looks like yours —
Because to me, you're the most beautiful person in this world.

And if I become a baby girl,
Can I look like Papa?
Because I know you love the way he smiles,
The way he stands strong beside you.
Maybe, then, you'll smile when you see me.

But Maa…
No matter what I become —
Boy or girl,
Soft or strong,
Curious or calm —
I want to say this…

I am only yours.
Born of your breath,
Held in your heartbeat.
I belong to your dreams, your hopes, your tears.

So Maa, will you still love me… if I am a girl?
Will you hold me with the same pride?
Will your eyes shine the same way when you see me?

Because I've heard whispers…
Of sorrow,
Of disappointment…
When a girl is born.

I don't understand, Maa.
Why do some parents hope only for boys?
Why do they feel something is missing when a girl comes?
Don't they know?
A girl can love deeper.
She can dream louder.
She can fly just as far.

Why do they think a baby girl can't do everything?
Why, Maa?

Will you… think that way too?

Please don't.
Please don't turn your face away if I'm not what the world expected.

Because I've heard your heartbeat from the inside…
And it never sounded like rejection.
It sounded like home.

Mother:
Oh my child…
Forgive this world.
Forgive its broken thoughts and tired traditions.
You are mine —
And I don't need to know your gender
To love you with everything I have.

Boy or girl,
You are my miracle.
You are the soul I prayed for.
And when you arrive…
I will hold you close
And whisper into your tiny ear:

"You are wanted. You are perfect. You are enough."

Mother's Diary Entry:

Dear Love,
I can feel you now —
Your tiny heart racing with questions I'm still too scared to ask myself.
You want to know if I'll love you if you're a girl,
And I can't help but wonder…
How have we, as a society, made even the purest souls like you question their worth,
Simply because of what they are born as?

If I could, I would hold you close now and tell you this:
It doesn't matter, my darling.
I will love you in ways the world has never learned to.
Whether you are a boy or a girl,
You are everything I've dreamed of —
Not just for who you will be,
But for who you already are to me.

There are things about this world I can't change,
The way people think,
The way they judge,
But I promise you,
I will never see you as anything less than perfect.
Not because of your gender,
But because of the love you will give,
The dreams you will chase,
The person you will become.

My love for you will never be based on expectations.
You are mine —
No matter what.
And I will hold you,
Tell you you're beautiful,
And show the world the kind of strength that runs through our veins —
The strength of unconditional love.

I can't wait to meet you, my child.
And when I do,
I will tell you this over and over:

You are wanted.
You are enough.
And you are loved beyond measure.

With all my heart,
Your Maa

"Mother's Diary"

My Dearest Love,
I have been thinking about your words all day long…
The way you asked, "Maa, will you still love me if I'm a girl?"
And I can't help but wonder —
Why, my baby, would you ever feel unsure of that?

Is it because of the world?
The world that sometimes doesn't know how to cherish the most delicate and powerful things in it?
The world that still believes some things are more valuable than others because of what they appear to be?
Oh, my little one, I wish I could shield you from that.

You are **my everything** —
Before you even had a body, before you had a name,
I loved you beyond measure.
I loved you the day I found out about you,
I loved you before I could even hear your heartbeat,

And I will love you the day I hold you in my arms,
Whether you are a boy or a girl.

If you are a girl, I will show you the strength of a woman who defies the expectations of this world.
I will teach you that your worth is not in what others see, but in what you feel inside — your dreams, your heart, your mind.
I will hold you and tell you that there's nothing you cannot do,
That you can conquer anything, and your worth is immeasurable.
You are not less. You are not limited.
You are everything this world needs and more.

If you are a boy, I will teach you to respect women —
To always see them as equals,
To honor their strength, their love, their beauty.
I will raise you to understand that being a man is not about dominance,
But about kindness, compassion, and responsibility.
I will teach you that true strength lies in lifting others up.
I will teach you how to love with humility.

But whether you are a boy or a girl —
You are **my miracle**, my child,
And I will raise you to know one truth:
You are perfect.
You are whole.
You are loved just as you are.

No matter how the world may look at you,
You are more than enough.

When you ask if I will still love you if you are a girl,
I wonder, will the world teach you to question your worth?
But know this, my precious one —
I will love you fiercely,
As only a mother can.
And the world will never tell me otherwise.

One day, when you're older, you will see how strong women have always been.
I will show you the women who broke barriers, who made history, who loved with such power that no one could stop them.
And you will know, my love, that being a girl is not something to fear,
But something to be proud of.
You are everything this world needs.
And I will be here to remind you of that every day.

Until I hold you, my sweet one,
I'll keep dreaming of the day I'll see your face,
The day I'll hear you call me "Maa,"
And the day I can tell you,
You are loved. You are wanted.
And you are perfect.

With all the love I carry in my heart,
Your Maa.

Baby: "Maa, I heard you today, when the room was quiet and everything was still. Your thoughts felt like a lullaby, wrapping around me, comforting me. I could feel your heart — you were speaking without words, and I understood every part of you."

Mother: "You feel my silence, don't you, my love? It's the space where I dream of you, where I speak to you in ways the world doesn't hear. The quiet is where I find you, where you grow."

Baby: "Maa, I moved today. Just a little nudge, but it felt like a promise. A promise that one day, I will hold your hand, and we will walk through this world together. I don't need to see you to know you are here — I can feel you with every heartbeat."

Mother: "My love, I felt it. A little flutter, just for me. My heart skipped a beat, and I whispered your name into the air. Even though I can't hold you yet, you are here. You are real. And I can't wait to hold you."

Baby: "Maa, do you ever feel scared? Do you wonder if you'll be a good mother? Do you think I'll be okay? Sometimes, I feel the weight of the world around us — it's heavy, isn't it?"

Mother: "Yes, love, I am afraid. Afraid of not being enough. Afraid of the world's judgments. But then I think of you — your tiny heart, your tiny soul — and I know that we will be okay. We are strong because we have each other. You will be everything this world needs, and I will be here to help you find your strength."

The Mother Reflecting on Her Own Journey and Hopes for Her Child

Mother: "I used to think I needed to be someone different to succeed in this world — I thought my worth depended on meeting others' expectations. But then you came into my life. And now I realize... success means being true to who we are. It means loving unconditionally, being kind, and never losing sight of what matters. When you come into this world, I hope you remember this above all else: Be yourself. The world needs you — just as you are."

Trimester 3

"I'm Ready to Meet You"

The final stage, baby grows big, strong, and prepares for birth.

Medical/Developmental Highlights:

Weeks 27–32: Baby begins to **kick stronger**, respond to light & touch, **brain developing fast**.

Weeks 33–36: Baby gains weight, body fills out, **sleep-wake patterns form**.

Weeks 37–40: Full term. Baby positions for birth, **lungs mature**, ready to meet you.

Emotional angle from baby's voice:

> "I'm almost ready, Maa. I dream of your face, your arms… and calling you Maa for the very first time."

Chapter 1

"I Can Hear Your Lullabies"

Dear Maa,

Your voice...
It's no longer just a sound to me.
It's a warm blanket that wraps around my tiny heart.

When you hum those soft lullabies before falling asleep... I listen.
When you whisper my name with hope and wonder... I listen.
Even when you cry softly, hiding your tears from the world... I hear you, Maa.

Inside you, the world is muffled, like being underwater — but your voice travels through everything, like light through the clouds. Your laughter makes me kick with joy. Your sobs... they make me curl tighter, wanting to comfort you from within.

You don't know this, but every time you touch your belly and say, "Baba will be home soon,"
I smile inside.
Because I know... I am loved by both.

And those lullabies you sing?
Someday, I will fall asleep in your arms while you sing the same ones — not through skin and heartbeat, but through touch and closeness.

I'm growing, Maa. I'm almost ready.
But for now, I'm just listening.
To you.
To love.
To life.

Dear Maa,

Do you know what your touch feels like from here?
Like moonlight brushing over a sleepy river...
gentle, calming, magical.

When your hands rest on your belly, I feel them.
When you rub me softly, as if saying "I'm here, baby",
I nuzzle back, as if saying "I feel you too, Maa."

Every time you place your warm palm and whisper,
"Are you okay in there?" —
I stretch a little, kick a little,
Just to let you know — yes, I'm okay. And I know you're there.

Your touch tells me stories.
It tells me when you're tired... when you've had a hard day...
But it also tells me when you're smiling while

thinking about me,
dreaming of the moment we'll finally meet.

And when Baba sends his love through your belly,
Or Dida gently rests her hand and talks to me,
I feel the warmth of a family already wrapped
around me like a blanket of love.

Maa, your touch isn't just physical —
It's spiritual.
It's a soft echo of the bond we've shared since the
first cell of me began to exist inside you.

I may not see the world yet,
But through your touch…
I already know what love feels like.

Chapter 2

"I Know Your Touch, Maa"

"Maa, your hands... I know them now."

When you gently rub your belly, I feel it. I sense the warmth in your palm, the softness in your touch. And I respond, don't I? With a tiny kick... or a little roll. It's my way of saying, "I'm here, Maa."

Every time your hand rests on your belly, I feel safer. It's like your love travels through your skin and reaches me directly. I may be small, but your touch is the biggest comfort I know.

"Do you feel me move when you touch me? That's me reaching out to you, in my own little way."

You often rest your hands on me when you talk, sing, or even cry softly at night. I know every feeling that flows through you, Maa. Your happiness fills me like sunlight, and your tears make me want to hold you back.

"Sometimes, I press my tiny hand or foot where I feel yours. Do you notice that, Maa?"

That's our little game, our silent language. You don't need words — just your gentle hand, and I understand everything. You're teaching me love even before I open my eyes.

So, keep touching, keep feeling, keep loving.
Because Maa...

"Your touch is my first lullaby, my first hug, my first world."

Chapter 3

"Your Dreams, My Future"

Dear Maa,

I don't dream yet…
But I live inside your dreams.
You whisper them to me — softly, lovingly —
As if painting my future with your hopes.

You talk about holding me close…
About dressing me in soft clothes,
About kissing my tiny fingers and watching me sleep like a little angel.
I may be floating here in the dark,
But your dreams are the light that guide me.

You wonder who I'll become.
Will I be strong? Kind? Smart?
Will I love books or music, or maybe stars and machines?
Maa, your every wish becomes a seed in my heart —
And one day, I will bloom with the flowers of your prayers.

I hear you say,
"I want to give you everything I couldn't have."
And even before I take my first breath,
You've already given me everything that matters —
Your love. Your strength. Your belief in me.

I may be your dream come true…
But Maa, your dreams are shaping who I will become.

Your voice is my guide.
Your wishes are my direction.
Your dreams… they are my future.

Chapter 4

"Counting the Days With You"

Dear Maa,

I don't know how to read clocks or calendars,
But I can feel it...
Every day, your heartbeat beats with more excitement.
Every night, your voice holds more hope.
You're counting the days, and so am I.
In my own tiny way.

The space around me is growing tighter,
Not uncomfortable — just... snug.
Like the universe is gently preparing me to leave the stars
and step into your arms.

Sometimes you talk to me while folding clothes,
Sometimes you pack my little things,
And sometimes... you pause, place your hand on your belly,
And whisper, "Just a few more weeks, my love."

Maa, I hear it in your breath.
In your tired feet, in your soft sighs,
And in that little tremble in your voice
when you say "I can't wait to hold you."

I want you to know…
I feel the same.
I can't wait to see your eyes.
To feel your skin against mine.
To hear your lullaby without the cushion of water and skin.
To breathe in the scent of my Maa.

Let's count these days together —
Not with numbers, but with love.
Because every day we get closer,
Is a day closer to forever.

Chapter 5

"Your Strength is My Shield"

Dear Maa,

I've heard people say, "Mothers are strong."
But they don't know just how strong you really are.
Because I do.
I live in your strength every day.

Every ache you bear,
Every restless night,
Every moment you feel breathless —
You still smile. You still whisper to me, "We're okay, baby."
And that's when I know…
Your strength is not just physical. It's made of love, stitched with courage.

When the world gets too loud,
Your steady heartbeat calms me.
When you feel weak,
You still hold on for me — like a warrior with a gentle soul.
Maa, you carry me…
Not just in your womb, but in your spirit.

Your worries, your silent tears,
your swollen feet, your tired back —
I feel them, Maa.
But I also feel your power.
And it shields me like armor made of devotion.

One day, when I open my eyes and see you for the first time,
I'll recognize you not just as my mother…
But as my first protector.
My first home.
My first hero.

Until then, I'll keep growing under the safety of your love —
The strongest shield in the universe.

Chapter 6

"Maa, I'm Coming"

Dear Maa,

Can you feel it?
Something is changing —
The world inside is no longer as quiet…
The space is tighter, your heart beats faster, and
your hands linger a little longer on your belly.

I know what this means.
It means it's almost time.
Time for me to leave the only world I've ever
known —
To enter yours.

I feel your excitement…
But I also feel your fear.
Your prayers have become whispers of strength,
Your thoughts are filled with questions,
And your eyes—yes, even through your skin—I feel
them shining with waiting.

Maa, I may be tiny,
But I carry your love like a lantern inside me.
It will guide me through the darkness.
Through the pain.
Through the unknown.
To you.

I don't know what light looks like yet.
I don't know how cold the air will feel.
But I know one thing —
Your arms will be there.
Your eyes will be the first thing I see.
Your voice, the first I truly understand.

And when you cry with joy,
As they place me on your chest…
I'll know — I'm home.

So hold on, Maa.
I'm gathering all my courage.
Just a little longer.
I'm coming to meet you.
To complete our journey… and begin another.

Chapter 7

"Afterword: My First Three Months in This New World"

Maa...
I was so safe inside you. You were my whole world — my sky, my earth, my everything. I felt your heartbeat, your warmth, your love. In your womb, I knew only comfort and calm.

But then, one day, I entered a new world — so vast, so bright, so loud... and so unknown.
I didn't know where I was. Everything felt infinite, unfamiliar, and overwhelming.
I couldn't express it, Maa, but I was afraid.

I didn't know how to tell you when I was cold.
Or when I felt hot.
When I had pain in my tiny body.
Or when I needed sleep, or food, or just your gentle touch.

I didn't know how to ask — I still don't.
I can't speak yet, but I feel everything.
I feel your presence, your love, your care — and that's what keeps me strong.

So please, Maa… keep me close.
Hold me gently. Watch over me, even when I'm sleeping.
Wrap me in your warmth until I can understand this world.
Protect me until I can protect myself.
Speak to me, love me, comfort me — until I can find the words to speak back.

Because even though I'm here now, outside of you…
You are still my universe.

Made in United States
Cleveland, OH
28 July 2025